HERBS FOR HEADACHES AND MIGRAINE

A practising medical herbalist explains the causes of headaches and migraine, gives dietary advice and describes, as well as showing how to use, twenty-one herbs that are helpful in relieving these distressing complaints.

By the same author
HERBS FOR COLDS AND FLU'
HERBS FOR THE HEART AND CIRCULATION

HERBS FOR HEADACHES AND MIGRAINE

by

NALDA GOSLING
F.N.I.M.H., M.B.N.O.A., N.D., D.O.

Drawings by A.R. Gosling

THORSONS PUBLISHERS LIMITED
Wellingborough, Northamptonshire

First published 1978
Second Impression 1980

ISBN 0 7225 0396 2

Photoset by
Specialised Offset Services Ltd., Liverpool
and printed and bound in Great Britain by
Weatherby Woolnough, Wellingborough, Northants

CONTENTS

MAKING A HERBAL INFUSION

Unless otherwise stated in the text, the normal method of making an infusion applies to each herb and is as follows: $\frac{1}{2}$ litre (1 pint) of boiling water is poured over 25g (1 oz.) of the dried herb, preferably in a warmed container, covered, and allowed to stand for fifteen minutes.

Roots of plants should be prepared by using the same quantities, adding the chopped root to cold water, bringing to the boil and simmering gently until reduced by one quarter, keeping a lid on the pan the whole time. Cool and strain.

The dose, unless included in the instructions, will be a wineglassful three times daily. A wineglassful is approximately equivalent to three tablespoonsful.

INTRODUCTION

Headaches and migraine are as old as man himself. The earliest written records date back to about 3,000 BC and many of the great physicians such as Hippocrates and Galen discussed causes and treatment. Galen (130-200 AD) was the first to use the name 'hemicrania' to describe migraine, which has been called such names as 'sick headache' and 'heterocrania', with spellings ranging from maigram to mygrim.

A headache is the most common symptom for which medical help is sought. Approximately 70 per cent of the population suffer from headaches, some only occasionally and others frequently, varying in degree from a slight, transient ache to an incapacitating pain. Only a few headaches are caused by serious disease; the majority are either tension headaches or of psychosomatic origin. The most common treatment is aspirin or some other analgesic (a drug to relieve pain). Two thousand tons of aspirin are swallowed in Britain each year (*British Medical Journal*, July 1974), and the tranquillizers librium and valium are the most commonly prescribed drugs. Such treatment will afford temporary relief but does not deal with the cause.

What is the approach of the herbal practitioner? He or she is naturally concerned with relieving pain, but mainly with ascertaining the cause and with directing the treatment toward that as a means of effecting a cure. Each patient is treated as an individual, and the approach is that of taking careful details of the health history, carrying out a thorough examination, systematically dealing with causes of ill-health and with improving the patient's general standards of health. There are over fifty herbs that are valuable for headaches, from which the practitioner may select the appropriate remedies for each patient and supplement their action with scores of others, varying them as required during the course of treatment.

The herbs discussed in this book are merely tokens of the wide range available for the treatment of headaches and migraine. Causes are discussed, dietetic measures are advised and a chapter is devoted to migraine.

Herbal remedies have been thoroughly tested by long usage and research, and normally they will be effective for the conditions described. However, certain serious organic illnesses give rise to headaches, so if no improvement is experienced after following the advice carefully, or if headaches are increasing, it would be wise to seek professional help.

1.

CAUSES

The actual pain of a headache or migraine is caused, in 90 per cent of cases, either by inflammation and swelling of blood vessels in the head, or by continuous spasm and contraction of neck muscles. The background causes which lead to this physical state are numerous. It must not be forgotten that a headache may be one of the first symptoms of an acute infection such as a cold or influenza. A dull or neuralgic headache with feverish symptoms, aching limbs or a feeling of chilliness could therefore be quickly treated and cleared by resting in a warm bed and drinking hot infusions of herbal teas such as Lime blossom, Elderflowers and Peppermint, Yarrow, or Composition Essence to promote perspiration.

Localized causes of headaches may be sinusitis or nasal catarrh, usually worse in the morning but easing during the day and returning later when the patient is fatigued, for which Eyebright taken as a warm infusion would be useful, or Anemone as a cool tea.

Eyestrain is an obvious cause of headaches across the forehead, with aching eyes, which develop after close work or during late afternoon and which hardly appear during holidays or weekends. In addition to the obvious points such as correct lighting, relaxing the eyes from time to time during the work, and carrying out eye exercises, either Eyebright or Rue may be used in cold infusion as an eyebath. To prepare the Eyebright, boil 25g (1 oz.) of herb in $\frac{1}{2}$ litre (1 pint) water for one minute, allow to stand for half an hour and strain through a fine cloth. Use this both in an eyebath and as a compress over the eyes and across the forehead, applying it for up to half an hour. Elderflowers may be used in the same way, and are prepared by simmering gently for five minutes and infusing for ten.

Tension and Worry

A great number of headaches are the result of tension in the muscles of neck and shoulders, and for this cause any of the remedies for nerves and tension listed in the index will be helpful; the combination of Scullcap, Valerian, Mistletoe and Wood Betony, in equal parts, will give relief, together with gentle massage of the muscles.

A simple – and obvious – cause of a dull headache may be lack of sleep, which itself may be due to anxiety, an over-active brain, overwork, or a too-hectic social life. Herbal teas and baths at bedtime of Hops, Lime flowers or Rosemary will be of great assistance in promoting a relaxation of mind and body, but the original reason for the insomnia, if such it is, should be dealt with.

Worry and anxiety may have a serious background of problems but a regime directed toward improving general health by good nutrition, relaxation and herbal teas such as Wood Betony or Passion flower alone, or Scullcap, Valerian, Vervain and Ladies Slipper in equal parts, one teaspoonful to a teacup of boiling water taken at bedtime, will aid the ability to resolve problems. Lack of sleep due to too much mental activity such as is experienced by a person engaged in studies or other brain work can be ameliorated by an infusion of Rosemary or Scullcap taken at bedtime.

Disorders that Cause Headaches

Many headaches are due to constipation or to liver or kidney disorders, and into this category come 'bilious headaches'. There are many herbal remedies for this type of headache, ranging from simple aperients such as Senna (between five and ten of the pods should be soaked overnight in a cupful of water, with a pinch of powdered Ginger added, and the liquid taken before breakfast); Dandelion, which will have a beneficial effect on both liver and kidneys; herbs for the liver such as Black Root, Barberry bark, Balmony, Centaury and Fringe Tree bark; or diuretics such as Buchu, Clivers, Wild Carrot, Parsley Piert, and many others for the kidneys. Any of these herbs may be taken alone or used in combination with others for greater effectiveness. For example, equal quantities of Dandelion root, Barberry bark, Agrimony, and Centaury, 25g (1 oz.) of the mixed herbs to $\frac{1}{2}$ litre (1 pint) of water, simmered gently for ten minutes, will influence liver function and assist digestion if one small wineglassful is taken after each meal; equal amounts of Dandelion, Buchu, Wild Carrot and Pellitory-of-the-Wall, prepared as above but simmered for only two or three minutes, and taken between meals, will be beneficial to both kidneys and liver.

It is advisable, with headaches of this nature, to pay attention to diet by increasing salads, vegetables and fresh fruit, by including roughage such as bran or muesli at breakfast-time and such fruits as prunes, figs and raisins for constipation, and by reducing fried foods and dairy products for the 'bilious headache'.

Menstrual Tension

Many of the headaches from which women suffer are associated either with the menstrual period or with nervous tension. Some of the remedies for these are included, and are listed in the index, each with its specific use. For example, Anemone is valuable for a headache which occurs when the period is light, Melilot for a throbbing headache with painful periods or during the menopause, and so on. Each of these remedies will gently assist the flow of the periods.

Menstrual headaches may be due to slight anaemia, lack of calcium or to hormone imbalance. Herbal remedies can be of assistance, supported by dietetic measures. For the anaemia Dandelion is a useful remedy, with equal amounts of Nettles, Vervain and Comfrey leaves: 25g (1 oz.) to $\frac{1}{2}$ litre (1 pint) cold water, simmered for ten minutes and allowed to cool. A small wineglassful should be taken about half an hour before each meal. Foods which contain iron should be increased (see section on diet).

There is a wide range of herbs for nervous tension, and considerable benefit will be found by taking any of these regularly. Good nutrition is of great importance when there is a tendency to nervousness, hysteria or irritability.

High Blood-Pressure

Headaches may be one of the symptoms experienced with high blood-pressure, although one authority claims that the headaches only appear after the patient has been told that his blood pressure is high! The headache usually starts at the back of the neck and extends upwards to the top. It may be throbbing and there may be an associated giddiness. Lime flower tea, Mistletoe or Melilot will be found helpful, and attention must be given to diet. There are different causes of raised blood pressure (hypertension) and if these herbal teas do not effect any improvement it would be wise to seek professional advice.

Hypoglycaemia

One cause of headaches which must not be overlooked is hypoglycaemia (low blood sugar). This is a condition about which there is increasing awareness and concern, and is regarded as one of the diseases of civilization. A great deal of research has been carried out in America, where the Hypoglycaemia Association Inc. has been formed to give advice on diet to hypoglycaemics. An American specialist has referred to it as 'a real health problem related to nutrition, environment and, to a lesser degree, heredity. It is a problem of civilization with stress as a way of life.'

Hypoglycaemia arises as a result of a high intake of refined carbohydrates (starches and sugars), which constantly stimulate the secretion of insulin to reduce blood sugar level; a constant intake of carbohydrates in excess of other foods leads to over-production of insulin which, together with the effect of stress on the adrenal glands, leads to an imbalanced state.

The symptoms are exhaustion after the least effort, headache, giddiness, trembling, perhaps nausea, craving for sweet foods, and irritability, which can clear quickly after a meal or a snack. Blood sugar rises quickly after taking a sweetened drink, a snack or a meal, but may fall equally rapidly if the food consisted mainly of carbohydrates. The typical headache of this condition is present on waking, with a feeling of fatigue, especially if no supper was taken the previous night. The headache will also appear during the morning or if there is a long interval between meals. A herbal practitioner will provide medicines for this condition, and will also give instructions on diet.

Psychogenic Headaches

Some authorities consider that up to 90 per cent of headaches are of nervous or psychogenic origin, meaning that there is no physical disorder or disease present. Psychologists suggest that a headache may develop – from unconscious motivation – as the result of an unresolved problem, or to enable the sufferer to escape from an unpleasant situation, or to gain sympathy or attention. Some severe headaches may be the result of suppressed anger or resentment, and cases have been quoted in which the headaches disappeared when the anger was expressed harmlessly. There is one case on record of a migraine subject being advised by her physician to take up some form of sport to work off her anger and resentment. She took up tennis, became a champion and was completely free from migraine.

Stress

Headaches may also be the result of stress, which can be physical, mental or emotional. A Canadian physician, Dr Hans Selye, undertook intensive studies on the effect of stress on the body, describing the stimulation of adrenal gland action, leading to increased heart action, release of stored glycogen (sugar), dilatation of the pupils of the eyes and raised blood pressure, all part of the 'fight or flight' reaction to combat stress. This complex reaction returns to normal when the stressful situation is over, and body equilibrium is maintained.

However, if the stress is repeated and continued over a long time – for example, in a quarrelsome marriage partnership or with difficult work-colleagues – the blood pressure may remain raised or adrenal glands become exhausted, symptoms such as headaches, irritability, fatigue and digestive disturbances will occur, poor assimilation of food and uncertain appetite may follow, leading to faulty nutrition, and a vicious circle of events is instigated.

In this type of situation the cause must be understood and dealt with, by talking over the problems with a wise friend or professional counsellor, and by undertaking a regime of building up general health and resistance to stress. Herbal teas such as Passion flower, Wood Betony, Vervain and Scullcap will have a soothing and relaxing effect; sound nutrition should include wheatgerm, green vegetables, adequate protein and all the vitamins, especially vitamin C and pantothenic acid.

Muscle tension builds up as a result of, or as an expression of, nervous tension, and it is essential that relaxation is learned and practised daily. In his book *Release from Nervous Tension*, Fink states: 'We must begin by learning the technique and habit patterns of muscular relaxation. This is the first step to health ...' Dr Hans Selye, in discussing stress, states that nothing is accomplished by telling people not to worry, but that they must find something to put in the place of the worrying thoughts. Trying concentration on pleasant thoughts, or some strenuous work, or even becoming involved in another person's worry, has often been found to put the problem into proportion.

Headaches Resulting from Injuries

Many chronic headaches are the result of injuries sustained from sports such as horse-riding, or from car accidents, and are caused by impacted or displaced vertebrae. Concussion following accidents may make headaches develop and create a number of symptoms due to inactivity of nerves in the neck. The headaches may be quite violent across the forehead and on top of the head and may occur as a result of coughing or sneezing. There can be depression, apathy, lack of concentration, insomnia, and almost a change of personality from energetic to inactive. Osteopathic treatment can in almost all of these cases correct such conditions.

Yet another structural cause of headaches, though not a common one, is a one-sided contraction of neck muscles following acute torticollis (wry-neck). This condition normally arises from a spasm of muscles on one side of the neck, which makes turning of the head extremely painful. If it is not correctly treated initially, a lessened degree of muscle contraction remains, giving rise to headaches perhaps months later.

Herbalists have many herbs which are prepared for use as lotions or liniments to treat painful conditions, and these are used in conjunction with internal medication and local massage or manipulation.

Severe and increasing headaches may indicate a serious organic disease. If no relief is found from correct application of any of the remedies or measures advised, therefore, professional diagnosis must be sought.

2.

DIET

Correct nutrition, whilst not being the complete answer in every case, will certainly contribute to relief from chronic headaches and migraine. The experience of naturopathic practitioners is that a good balanced diet will not only improve general health and provide more vitality, but – when specifically planned – will reduce the main symptoms and conditions of which the patient complains.

A diet which includes fresh whole foods, adequate protein, fats, vitamins and minerals, a minimum of carbohydrates, and which excludes processed refined foods, should be followed.

Breakfast

Breakfast may consist of fruit juice (fresh, if possible, otherwise frozen or tinned unsweetened juice); fruit, either fresh, or dried stewed fruit such as prunes and apricots; wholewheat cereal or muesli; some form of protein; and yogurt if desired. The type of breakfast you have is the foundation for the day. If you have little time, a good muesli, with wheatgerm, seedless raisins, grated apple and skimmed milk powder added, together with milk, nut cream or soya milk substitute, will be more nutritious than refined cereals.

People who have no appetite in the morning would be well advised to take a course of herbal teas for the liver and digestion. To create a healthy appetite, make a tea by simmering 25g (1 oz.) Fringe Tree bark for ten minutes in 1 litre (2 pints) water, pour this on to 12g ($\frac{1}{2}$oz.) each Agrimony and Meadowsweet, and take a wineglassful three times daily between meals. Alternatively simmer equal parts of Dandelion root and Gentian, to make 25g, for ten minutes in 1 litre of water and pour on to 25g Agrimony, add a pinch of powdered ginger and take a wineglassful before meals, or take an infusion of Agrimony, alone before meals.

Lunch
If the main meal of the day is taken in the evening, lunch should include salad. Any number of raw vegetables grated, shredded or chopped finely, may be added to the basic salad greens, celery, tomato and cucumber. Nuts and dates or raisins may be added, or chopped apple, orange segments, chopped pineapple, and fresh or dried herbs such as Chives, Parsley, Lovage, Fennel, young Dandelion or Comfrey leaves, and Nasturtium leaves, may be chopped and sprinkled over the salad to vary the flavour. Food should be delicious and should be enjoyed, as well as being wholesome. Protein should be eaten with the salad, and a baked jacket potato or homemade soup included in cold weather. Wholewheat bread or crispbreads may be taken, if becoming overweight is not a problem. Fruit or yogurt may follow.

For those who have to take the midday meal away from home, salad can be carried easily in a container with a well-fitting lid, and may simply consist of celery, tomato, watercress or other manageable greens. One nutritionist claimed that a completely balanced meal could be had by having a good helping of Cheddar cheese, watercress and wholewheat bread with butter.

Evening Meal
The evening meal will naturally be, for the majority

of people, a cooked meal of protein, whether it is meat (not pork), fish, fowl, vegetarian protein such as nut, cheese or egg dishes, or soya protein, with vegetables. The vegetables should be cooked conservatively – that is, baked or casseroled, or cooked for the minimum length of time in the minimum of water, and the water should be used, not thrown away. Green leafy vegetables should be taken each day (the dark leaves are a good source of vitamins A and C) and carrots for vitamin A; pulses are useful sources of protein, and root vegetables also have value.

A dessert of fresh or stewed fruit, or a prepared sweet consisting mainly of fruit is preferable to a stodgy pudding.

At bedtime, a drink of yeast extract (such as Marmite or Vecon), herbal teas as indicated by symptoms, or fruit juice may be taken. A snack is advised in cases of hypoglycaemia, for the reasons referred to on page 13. Tea and coffee should be kept to the minimum, taken weak, or avoided for specific conditions.

A Balanced Diet

This brief outline of diet cannot possibly cover all the aspects of sound nutrition. Basically, the regime should include raw fruits, salads and vegetables (some authorities recommend that at least 50 per cent of foods should be raw), whole cereals (81 per cent and 100 per cent flour, for all baking, unpolished rice instead of white, and other whole cereals), honey or brown sugar for sweetening, vegetable oils instead of animal fats, and adequate protein (the requirement varies with individuals). Food should be fresh and compost-grown as far as possible, and processed refined foods avoided. About 2,000 chemicals are used in the production of food, of which over 1,000 are flavouring agents. Other chemicals are used for colouring, preserving, emulsifying and stabilizing. There are warnings from time to time that a chemical has been found to present some hazard or to be toxic, and it is banned or its use limited. It is surely advantageous to limit the intake of chemicals to the minimum, because although they are all used in infinitesimal amounts, the total and cumulative effect cannot always be predicted.

Now to consider some suggestions on diet which are more specifically for the causes of headaches.

Sinusitis and Catarrh

In sinusitis and chronic nasal catarrh it is wise to reduce milk and cheese, particularly cutting out a milky drink at bedtime, and to increase vitamin C. This could be in the form of lemon juice in hot water at bedtime, or as a controlled dose of about 500mg vitamin C in capsule form – Rose-hip, or something similar, is recommended. An infusion of Eyebright taken two or three times a day will be found helpful. Many cases of sinusitis have improved quickly as a result of taking both vitamin A and vitamin C.

Liver Conditions

Dairy products should also be reduced in liverish conditions. Many sufferers from migraine or chronic recurrent headaches experience a bad head after a meal containing cheese, eggs, milk or fats. Although these foods are required to provide a completely balanced diet, for the purpose of cure, it would be wise to avoid them as far as possible and at the same time to take remedies for the liver and digestive system. Herbs in this category are referred to on page 11 and in the Index.

Kidney Disorders and Constipation

Herbal practitioners have many remedies for the kidneys, and diet may have to be individually planned. Salt and coffee should be avoided, and the amount of protein will need adjustment. For constipation, roughage should be increased. The diet outlined above may provide enough roughage to cure the constipation; if not, it can be added to by taking, for a while, a tablespoonful or two of bran at breakfast time on muesli, into which a whole apple (including skin) has been grated. Prunes and figs should be taken at breakfast or a tablespoonful of washed seedless raisins soaked overnight in water and both fruit and water taken at breakfast.

High Blood-Pressure

When the blood pressure is raised alcohol and coffee must be eliminated from the diet entirely, and either Matté, Lime blossom or weak China tea taken. It would be wise to replace most of the animal protein with vegetarian proteins, and to increase vitamins B, C and E. Salt must be reduced. No more than three eggs per week should be eaten. Up to 300 units of vitamin E should be taken daily starting with a small dose and increasing gradually.

Nervous Disorders

Nervous disorders and nervous tension will benefit from the general diet outlined at the beginning of this chapter, with the addition of vitamins B and E and calcium. These three are present in whole cereals, but could be supplemented temporarily by taking Brewers Yeast tablets (three with each meal) and vitamin E capsules (a dose of 100-200 units daily). Yogurt will supply calcium and will also help to correct intestinal fermentation, as will Chamomile tea. As a point of interest, it was reported in *The Lancet* as long ago as 1966 that a Swedish doctor found improvement in eight out of ten migraine patients after giving them *Lactobacillus acidophilus*, which is present in yogurt. Yeast extract (such as Marmite and Vecon) as drinks, especially at bedtime, will benefit nervous conditions in many cases, as will many of the herbal teas (see *Therapeutic Index*). Coffee should be avoided because it has a stimulating effect on the nervous system with subsequent let-down. The repeated stimulus by taking several cups of coffee during the day is irritating to a nervous system which may be already over-stimulated by stress.

Hypoglycaemia

The diet in hypoglycaemia should consist of frequent meals or snacks which are high in protein content with some fat, and low in carbohydrates. White flour and white sugar should be avoided. A good breakfast containing protein is an essential in this condition. Research in America has shown that blood sugar – which provides energy – remains at a normal level for the greater part of the day after a substantial breakfast, whereas it drops sharply after a light breakfast of mainly starchy foods and only rises briefly after each intake of food during the remainder of the day.

Deficiency or Excess of Certain Nutrients

Many types of headaches and migraine are due to deficiencies of certain foods, or excess of others, and these respond to a change in nutrition. It has been found that lack of iron, of vitamin B, especially B1, B6 and B12, or of calcium, has contributed in many instances to recurrent headaches, and that adding these to the diet in adequate quantities has cleared the headaches permanently.

The headache and pre-menstrual tension which cause irritability and fatigue will respond quickly to vitamin D and calcium. A menstrual headache when there is iron deficiency will respond to wheatgerm and foods containing iron. Nettles, for example, are rich in iron, and the young leaves may be cooked in the same way as spinach and eaten as a vegetable. Young Dandelion leaves may be chopped and included in salad. It has been discovered that a pound of Dandelion leaves contains 163mg vitamin C, 61,970 i.u. vitamin A, 12.3g of protein, 14mg iron, 849mg calcium, in addition to other nutrients. A great number of wild plants are valuable sources of vitamins and minerals.

3

MIGRAINE

Migraine has been the subject of intense study for a very long time, the first comprehensive description – a vivid account – being by an eastern physician named Aretaeus in 90 AD, in which were detailed all the symptoms specific to this complaint. Many writers have subsequently added their descriptions, experiences and theories. Much research has been carried out, and literally thousands of papers written. One of the most searching studies in recent years was by Dr Harold Wolff of the New York Hospital, a work which is still an authority on the subject although it was published in 1963. More recently an excellent textbook has been written by Dr Oliver W. Sacks.

Classical Migraine
The major types of migraine are Classical and Common. Classical migraine may only last two or three hours, and hardly ever more than twelve hours, recurring after between two and ten weeks. The intense headache, affecting either side or both and developing into a deep, boring pain over one eye, is preceded by the aura, disturbances of vision lasting only a few minutes to an hour. The vision may be partly obliterated in one or both eyes by brilliant, contrasting zig-zags or other patterns, moving quickly or slowly, intense light or black and white. This aura usually clears as the headache develops. There may be sensory symptoms during the aura, temporary changes in touch, smell, hearing, or weakness of a limb, changes of mood, and

dreaminess as if in a trance. Classical migraine clears quickly, leaving the patient feeling well, energetic and alert.

Common Migraine

Common migraine, of which there are ten times more cases, lasts at least eight hours and often a whole day or longer, but will recur less regularly. The major symptoms are intense headache and nausea, with a variety of other symptoms such as drowsiness, irritability, stuffiness of the nose, light-headedness, abdominal pain and distension, pallor or redness of the face, sensitivity to light. The headache most frequently starts on one side of the head as a deep throbbing pain in the temple, and may remain there during the whole attack or may become more diffuse. Nausea is intense, with increased salivation and catarrh, and usually culminates in vomiting. There is a general feeling of discomfort, the patient has to lie down in a darkened room, and will feel exhausted for several days after the attack. Common migraine is usually ended either by vomiting or by a sound refreshing sleep.

Other Kinds of Migraine

Other types of migraine occur, such as menstrual migraine, which is self-evident. Circumstantial migraine occurs following such stimuli as certain foods (chocolate, cheese, milk, fats, fried foods), alcoholic drinks, intense or flickering light, noise, changes in climate, specific smells or perfumes, violent emotion or excitement, 'exercise or – conversely – rest, the latter being 'weekend migraine'.

Migrainous neuralgia, fortunately uncommon, was first described in 1867. The pattern is of a number of intense headaches of abrupt onset and always affecting the same side, occurring close together over a period of days or weeks, with a long interval between of months or years. The pain is excruciating and causes the patient to pace to and fro instead of lying down. One of the alternative names for this condition, which affects ten times more men than women, is 'cluster headache'.

Causes of Migraine

Theories of the causes of migraine have existed since the Greeks first propounded the 'humoral theory', that migraine was caused by bilious disturbances. There are three current theories: chemical, electrical and vascular. Each contains an element of truth, yet none completely explains the plethora of symptoms. Chemicals such as histamine, acetylcholine, sodium nitrite or the tyramine present in cheese and chocolate, have been found to precipitate headaches but not the complex of symptoms.

The electrical theory is that migraine is a disturbance of brain function, yet no clear pattern has emerged in spite of thirty years study using electroencephalogram measurement of brain activity on innumerable patients. This theory is not far removed from the nineteenth-century theory of 'nerve storms'. It has been verified that blood vessels dilate, become engorged with blood and thus cause head pain, but this phenomenon cannot be responsible for the wide range of symptoms.

There is no doubt that, in the majority of cases, psychological factors play a vital role. Some writers have described the 'migraine personality', an inflexible, ambitious, successful yet cautious perfectionist, well-controlled and therefore subject to outbursts (Wolff, 1963), or a person with repressed hostility (Fromm-Reichmann, 1937), or yet a person whose feelings of inadequacy lead to seeking attention, unconsciously, by means of illness. Such cases as these have a subconscious driving force which makes their migraine resistant to medicinal aid; therefore, an understanding and acknowledgement of the underlying emotional stresses and resolution of problems is essential. Psychosomatic migraine provides greater discussion than space will permit in this book, so the final conclusion must be that there is an innate tendency to migraine, 'the constitution of the nervous system' according to Darwin, together with an acquired pattern of symptoms due to environmental pressures, and migraine thus becomes a physical expression of feelings which the patient cannot voice.

According to different studies, about 50 per cent of migraine patients have either one or both parents who suffer from the condition. This does not prove genetic heredity, merely the influence of the emotional or dietetic pattern of family life. The cyclic vomiting of childhood has been noted as leading to migraine in later life. Migraine may begin in childhood, but about 40 per cent of the cases start after the age of thirty; menstrual migraine may occur during the whole of a woman's menstruating life, diminishing during the menopause. Recent evidence has shown that certain contraceptive pills have caused migraine in some women.

The Symptoms of Migraine

Fear is often expressed that the repeated pain and swelling of blood vessels may cause permanent damage. In thousands of cases of habitual migraineurs this has never been found to happen. Care must be taken not to confuse migraine with an inflammatory condition of blood vessels in the head, temporal arteritis. Pain can be in the temple or may be in the neck or even the jaw. The affected blood vessel is extremely tender to touch and may not pulsate. There is a general feeling of illness, possibly a raised temperature and varied aches and pains. If not treated quickly there is the danger of the inflammation spreading to the retinal artery supplying the eyes and to blindness. A headache of increasing severity over a period of weeks or months, with a feeling of pressure within the head could also indicate a serious condition and must demand professional attention.

How to Relieve It

How can one deal with migraine? From reading the preceding paragraphs, which provide but an abbreviated outline of this complex condition, it will be realized that there is no standard answer. Each person requires individual assessment and treatment. Medical herbalists and other practitioners of natural therapeutics can testify to the success of their methods, by which innumerable people have gained relief and cure from migraine.

The treatment must be systemic, not symptomatic: by dietetic measures (see section on diet), by attending to any psychosomatic cause and by taking herbal medicine consistently, with symptomatic treatment occasionally if required. A specific formula cannot be given, as the medicine must be an individual prescription. Although only four remedies are given in the therapeutic index, scores of others are used to supplement their action and to treat the causes and different stages of the condition.

It is essential to deal with stress, to avoid tense anticipation of the next attack, to cultivate a relaxed and philosophical attitude to life, remembering that migraine is not a malignant and fatal condition. Once the established pattern of migraine attacks has been broken, confidence will be gained, further improvement will take place and migraine will become but a vague memory.

4

ANEMONE
(Anemone pulsatilla)

This dainty plant grows extensively in northern and central Europe and western Asia, on dry soil. It is about 30 cm (12 inches) in height, and has a single dull purple flower with silky under-surface rising from a rosette of deeply-cut stalked leaves. It has grown wild in some parts of Britain, but is now rarely found. Its common names are Pasque flower, a name chosen by the great English herbalist, Gerard, because it blooms during April, or Windflower, perhaps for the graceful way it bows and moves in even the lightest breeze on the dry open slopes it favours.

The action of Anemone is sedative, analgesic and

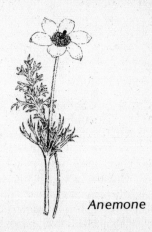

Anemone

nervine. It is one of the finest remedies for a headache due to tension, its soothing, calming effect being reinforced when combined with Passiflora. It is specific for headaches suffered by sensitive women of gentle or timid disposition, for headaches with pressure on the vertex (top of the head), with neuralgic pains which mostly affect the right side. It can be beneficial when the headache is associated with painful scanty menstruation, or is due to overwork in an over-active, highly emotional mental state.

An infusion may be made from the dried plant, the dose being one wineglassful three times daily, taken cold, or only occasionally as required for a headache, or at bedtime. The bedtime dose, if combined with Passiflora, will be conducive of calm refreshing sleep.

The tincture of Anemone is used by herbalists to relieve spasms of asthma, and is recommended as a regular medicine to clear catarrh, as it has an effect on all mucous membranes. Small doses are advisable.

5.

CHAMOMILE
Roman: (Chamaemelum nobile)
(Anthemis nobilis)
German: (Matricaria chamilla)

The Roman Chamomile, which has a pleasant aroma of apples, is cultivated extensively in several western European countries. Its scent probably led the Greeks to name it *kamai melon* 'ground apple'. Chamomile belongs to the *Compositae*, an extensive Order of plants which include about one-tenth of all known species of flowering plants. The flowers in

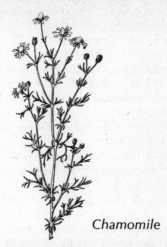

Chamomile

the Order consist of numerous small florets compounded together to form one flower, including such well-known plants as the common daisy, golden rod, groundsel, yarrow, and the sunflower. Many of the plants possess medicinal properties, and many produce beautiful flowers such as the dahlia. The chamomile grows naturally in Britain, on waste ground and heathland, but the flowerheads from the cultivated plant are used in medicine. The whole plant is bitter, owing to anthemic acid, its major constituent being a volatile oil.

The action of Chamomile is sedative, carminative and anti-emetic. Chamomile tea has long been known for its soothing effect on the nervous system, and for allaying nausea or the sickness of pregnancy. It is particularly beneficial for digestive disturbances with flatulence; in cold infusion the appetite is stimulated and digestion improved, in hot infusion it will relieve biliousness and promote perspiration in colds – for this a little ginger should be added.

This remedy should be used for headaches which occur during the menstrual period, when there is pain, irritability and scanty flow, but it is not advisable in heavy periods.

Chamomile has been found most effective for a bilious headache, relieving the nausea and relaxing tension. It is well known as a household remedy for childhood conditions: restlessness, colic, colds, measles, earache.

The infusion may be made by pouring $\frac{1}{2}$ litre (1 pint) of boiling water on to 25g (1 oz.) of the flowers, or by using four to eight flowers to a teacupful of boiling water, sweetening with honey. The dose is a teaspoonful for infants or more according to age, to a small teacupful for headaches or nausea, taken two or three times daily as required. It may be taken warm for fevers or colds, when the dose should be small, and as a cold infusion for stomach disturbance, headaches and nervousness. A dose one hour before meals acts as an appetiser. This is a remedy for which claims of preventing nightmares have been made.

The German Chamomile is considered by some to be a more pleasant drink. The flowers are smaller than the Roman Chamomile, and the infusion is made with one teaspoonful of the flowers to a teacup of boiling water, allowed to infuse (covered) for three to five minutes – no longer – and strained. *Matricaria* may be used for similar conditions to those described above, but it is more specific for a restlessness and irritability, and for a throbbing headache which only seems to affect one part of the head. Taken after a meal it aids digestion.

The infusion strained through muslin or gauze is soothing as an eyebath or compress for inflamed eyes.

6

CORN SILK
Stigmata maidis (Zea mays)

Maize (corn) first became known to the western world in 1492, but had been the most important cereal in Mexico and South America long before then. Evidence indicates that it may have been established as a crop 5,000 years ago. Corn is a nutritious food which is low in gluten. The oil extracted from it is used widely for cooking and for making margarine. This oil is a good source of linoleic acid, which reduces blood cholesterol.

It has a unique structure in that the flowers are packed in rows along the cob, each flower producing a long Silk and one grain or seed. The Silk is the part used medicinally, and is a soothing

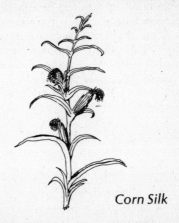

Corn Silk

diuretic which is valuable for all inflammatory conditions of the bladder and kidneys, especially for offensive, scanty urine which smells of ammonia, for acute or chronic cystitis, painful or slow urination, and a catarrhal state of the urinary system.

Corn Silk has an antiseptic action. It is effective in uric acid conditions either used alone or combined with Dandelion root. Take two parts of Corn Silk to one part of Dandelion root, chopped finely, infusing one teaspoonful of the mixture in a teacup of boiling water. Allow to stand for at least one hour. The mixture may be sweetened with a little honey if desired. Take this quantity three times daily.

Corn Silk has proved useful in cases of enuresis (bed-wetting), for which it is combined with Agrimony. Use in equal parts, adding one teaspoonful to a small teacup of boiling water and allowing to cool. Take at bedtime. If the tinctures are available, take ten drops of each in a little water morning and afternoon, between meals and at bedtime (a smaller dose for a child).

This remedy is useful for headaches which are associated with kidney and urinary conditions, and is prepared by adding half a tablespoonful of the dried Silk to one teacupful of cold water. Bring it almost to the boil, and keep on a very low heat for three minutes. Allow to cool and take once or twice daily as required.

7.

COUCH GRASS
(Agropyron repens)

A pest to gardeners and farmers, a boon to the herbal practitioner, Couch Grass grows extensively in Europe, America, Australia and parts of Asia. Its

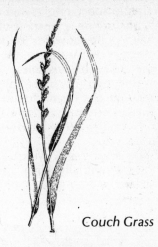

Couch Grass

name is from the Anglo-Saxon word *civice* 'vivacious', describing its tenacity to life. It increases both by creeping rootstock and by seed-dispersal, and a single plant has been known to produce 10,000 seeds. Unless it is pulled up completely in early spring it will increase more and more as it is cut.

This is a remedy to use for headaches due to disorders of the urinary system. It is one of the finest and most gently diuretic remedies for all conditions of kidneys and bladder, relieving irritation and inflammation and increasing the flow of urine. It relieves backache due to kidney disorder, is soothing in cystitis, especially when combined with buchu leaves, is a good remedy for gout and rheumatism, and has been found to exert its influence on the liver. Dioscorides recommended it for difficulty in passing urine, and Gerard said of it: 'Although that couch-grasse be an unwelcome guest to fields and gardens, yet his physick virtues do recompense ...'

The rhizome – the thickened stem which serves as

a creeping rootstock – is the part used. It is gathered in spring, cut into short lengths and dried. It should be prepared by adding a heaped tablespoonful to one and a half teacups of water, bringing to the boil and simmering gently for three minutes. Add a little liquorice, honey or molasses, allow to cool and take teacupful doses two or more times daily. Pre-menstrual tension and headaches are often due to fluid-retention; Couch Grass could therefore be taken as a preventative medicine during the few days before a period is due.

Couch Grass is a remedy which will bring quick relief and will eventually clear the symptoms if persisted with.

8.

DANDELION
(Taraxacum officinale)

Too well-known to need description, this common plant is disliked by gardeners, yet is beautiful in the construction of its flowers. A remedy known to the Greeks, who named it from *taraxos* 'disorder' *akos* 'remedy'. It played an important part in Arabian medicine, was esteemed by Gerard, Parkinson, and by many other reputable herbalists, and is an agent used most extensively by herbal practitioners. Dandelion possesses diuretic and laxative properties, and has long been known for its remarkable ability to increase the output of urine. The root has been the part used, but recent research is producing evidence of great value in the leaves, which contain 7,000 i.u. vitamin A per 25g (1 oz.), vitamins B and C, natural sodium, and active diuretic properties. The leaves are valuable in spring as one of the cleansing herbs which act as a tonic after winter. Young leaves

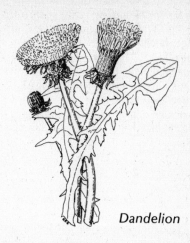

Dandelion

may be added to salads, or may be made into a tea (three teaspoonsful to a teacup of boiling water, covered and infused for ten minutes), or added to soups, providing a health-giving addition to the diet. A decoction may be made by soaking equal parts of chopped roots and leaves in cold water – 50g (2 oz.) to $\frac{1}{2}$ litre (1 pint) – for an hour, bringing gently to the boil, taking off heat and allowing to cool. Take one cupful before each meal.

Dandelion is combined with other remedies by the herbal practitioner for a variety of urinary conditions, for chronic constipation, dyspepsia and some liver conditions.

Recent scientific research shows that the remedy doubles the output of bile, confirming its use for liver and gastric disorders. This remedy should be used for the dull headache associated with bilious attacks or gastric disturbances, sluggish digestion and a muddy complexion. It may be taken as a tea, from fresh or dried leaf or root, or as a fluid extract (which is included in the British Pharmacopoea) with a dose of five to ten drops three times daily, according to laxative properties required. A valuable treatment for liverish headaches or migraine, which needs to be taken regularly over a period of weeks, is the following: 12g ($\frac{1}{2}$ oz.) each Dandelion root, Wild Carrot, Marshmallow root, Motherwort, Vervain and Ginger root. Mix together and put half the quantity into 1 litre of water, bring to the boil and simmer very gently for fifteen minutes. The dose is a half teacupful three times daily before meals.

9.

FEVERFEW
(Chrysanthemum parthenium)

Both English and Latin names of this plant ascribe to its virtues, 'few' from the Latin *fugo* 'put to flight', and 'parthenium' which is one of the names of the Greek goddess Athene, who, in mythology according to Pliny, outlined its medicinal properties to Pericles. A member of the *Compositae*, a Natural Order amounting to about 10,000 species, this plant grows fairly profusely in hedgerows and on waste ground. It is recognizable by its many white flowers and finely-cut delicate green leaves which gave rise to its other name, Featherfew. It is pleasantly aromatic, although the perfume is said to be disliked by bees.

It has long been used in warm infusion for fevers, and was valued so highly that Gerard claimed that the leaves fastened around the wrists would prevent ague.

One of the most widely known uses is for women's ailments, to help aid the flow of menstruation, for nervous hysteria at period time, for hot flushes during the menopause, and as a general tonic. It is

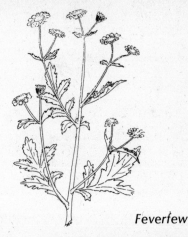

Feverfew

used for headaches which occur at the period, when the regularity is disturbed, causing an ache on the top of the head. The normal infusion should be prepared, and taken in a dose of two tablespoonsful night and morning, or when required for a headache.

10.

GENTIAN
(Gentiana lutea)

The yellow gentian, a plant which grows at high altitudes in southern and central Europe, was named after King Gentius of Illyria, who, according to Pliny, discovered its considerable medicinal virtues.

It is stimulating to the appetite and digestion, and is the remedy to use for a dull headache across the forehead, perhaps with dizziness, and with lack of appetite, nausea and dyspepsia. A decoction may be

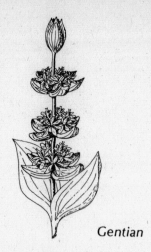

Gentian

made by simmering 25g (1 oz.) of the finely cut root in ½ litre (1 pint) of water for fifteen minutes, allowing it to cool. The dose is two teaspoonsful before meals. It may be sweetened slightly with honey, or such pleasant herbs as Peppermint, Balm or Lime blossom added for the benefit they provide and for the flavour. This herb is used by the herbal practitioner in combination with other herbs for biliousness, indigestion, general debility, exhaustion after prolonged illness, for headaches due to disorder of the digestive system, and it is used to reinforce the action of such nervines as Scullcap, Valerian, Vervain, and Mistletoe for nervous exhaustion. It has been found to ease prolonged vomiting. It increases the flow of saliva and digestive juices, and improves the appetite.

The root is the part used, and as appreciation of its value has increased the wild plant is being depleted to such an extent that cultivation is becoming necessary.

HOPS
(Humulus lupulus)

The beautiful climbing plant is more widely known for its use in making beer than for its medicinal values, yet it has been used for about 1,000 years, was known to the Romans and written about by Pliny. The Romans were fond of it as a vegetable: the young shoots are not unlike asparagus. Although it may be found growing wild in hedgerows it was introduced to Britain from Holland in about 1524 for beer-making. Its Latin name, *Humulus*, is derived from the Old Dutch word 'hommel'.

The plant contains a volatile oil which is used in perfumery, and bitter principles. It is sedative and is an excellent nervine. The catkin – strobile – is the

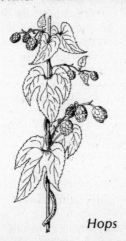

Hops

part used, and may be made into an infusion using 12g (½ oz.) to ½ litre (1 pint) of boiling water, allowing it to infuse for ten minutes. Do not allow any steam to escape. A wineglassful may be taken three times daily; taken before meals it acts as a tonic in exhaustion and debility, taken after meals it improves the digestion. This remedy is for headaches or neuralgia associated with nervous tension and restlessness, especially with insomnia due to nervous irritation. A cupful of the tea, which may be the above infusion or three teaspoonsful of crushed strobiles to a teacupful of boiling water, taken at bedtime, will calm the nerves, ease a headache, and if taken regularly will prevent unpleasant dreams or nightmares. In addition, a bath which contains 25g (1 oz.) of hops in a muslin bag, or a small pillow stuffed with hops will quickly help to cure insomnia.

Hops, used in tincture, fluid extract or infusion, have been used by herbalists for a variety of conditions, possessing properties which check the increase of bacteria, improve the function of liver and gall bladder, increase gently the flow of urine, relieve some irritating skin conditions and relieve neuralgic pains. The remedy would not be used by the herbalist for a melancholy or depressed patient, but in restlessness and excitability.

Hops may be used externally as a poultice for painful swellings, neuralgia, boils and abscesses.

12.

LAVENDER
(Lavendula vera)

This familiar garden plant needs no description. Containing from 1.5 to 3 per cent volatile oil, it grows wild on dry mountainous slopes in the

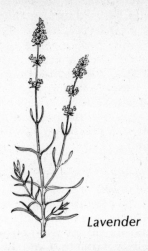

Lavender

Mediterranean lands, and is cultivated extensively for use in perfumery in France, Italy and many other countries. English lavender has been claimed to produce the finest oil, 27kg (60 lbs) of flowers yielding about 400g (16 oz.) of oil.

Known to the Greeks who named it Nardus, mentioned by St Matthew as Spikenard, used abundantly by the Romans as a perfume in the bath, and in other European countries for strewing churches on festive occasions, it has been widely used throughout the ages, both aromatically and medicinally.

Lavender is sedative, carminative, antiseptic, and is a fine nerve tonic. The essential oil has been proved by modern research to be a powerful antiseptic, verifying its application in the past to heal wounds or insect bites. One to three drops of the oil on sugar will quickly relieve headaches, faintness or giddiness, palpitation, colic, or a little of the oil may be rubbed on the temples to relieve a nervous headache. A weak infusion may be made from 6g

($\frac{1}{4}$ oz.) of the flowering tops in 1 litre (2 pints) of boiling water, infused for five minutes (do not allow the steam to escape), taken in teacupful doses between meals, two or three times daily, will be soothing and have a sedative action on the whole nervous system. An oil may be made by putting a handful of fresh flowers in a glass jar, covering with olive oil and leaving to stand in the sunshine for three days. Strain through a cloth, add fresh flowers and repeat the process until the oil is well-perfumed, when it will be ready for use. Four or five drops of this oil each day may be taken on sugar, and has been found very effective for migraine, dizziness, and nervous digestive disorders.

Lavender has been officially recognized in the British Pharmacopea since early in the eighteenth century, and its virtues were claimed: 'against the Falling-sickness, (epilepsy) and all cold Distempers of the Head, Womb, Stomach and Nerves; against the Apoplexy, Palsy, Convulsions, Megrim (migraine), Vertigo, Loss of Memory, Dimness of Sight, Melancholy ... It is an excellent but costly medicine'.

13.

LIME
(Tilia europoea)

The flowers of *Tilia europoea*, a native British tree, which perfume the surrounding air in early summer, are sedative and antispasmodic, and provide the herbalist with a fine remedy for migraine. They have proved their effectiveness in reducing nervous tension and lowering high blood pressure, either in the form of infusion, tincture or fluid extract. They may be combined with an equal quantity of Hops as

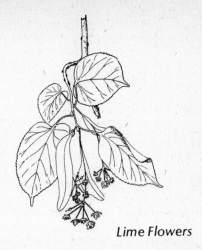

Lime Flowers

a cool infusion for tension and sleeplessness.

Taken alone in infusion during an attack of migraine, Lime flower tea will relax the blood vessels in the head, thus reducing pain, and will help allay nausea and vomiting. Passing a good quantity of urine can help reduce pressure on blood vessels, and here the diuretic properties of Lime flowers can prove effective.

Infusion of Lime flowers is helpful in relieving the dull headache which results from lack of sleep, and obviously in this instance should be taken regularly at bedtime to establish normal healthy sleep.

This remedy is also useful in headaches with neuralgia, which tend to affect first the right then the left side, and in which vision is affected.

Lime flower tea has diaphoretic properties when taken hot, and will quickly help to clear a cold in the early stages, especially when combined in equal parts with Elderflowers.

A wineglassful of the infusion taken after meals will aid digestion.

14

MELILOT
(Melilotus officinalis)

This dainty plant, with its spikes of yellow flowers arranged along one side of its stems, is a member of the *Leguminosae*, a Natural Order of about 6,500 species found in almost all parts of the world, ranging from tiny plants to massive trees, and including foods such as peas and beans, trees such as Rosewood and Acacia, Balsam of Peru, Mimosa, and the Manna mentioned in the scriptures.

Melilot is a remedy to use for a throbbing headache, with a feeling of fullness in the head which may be associated either with the menstrual period or with high blood pressure. It is also beneficial in a sick headache, where there is nausea or vomiting.

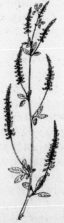

Melilot

Use this remedy when the hands and feet are cold,
but with throbbing and heat in the head.

An infusion of 40g (1½ oz.) to 1 litre (2 pints) should
stand for fifteen minutes, and the cool tea be taken
in wineglassful doses three or four times daily.

The ancient Egyptians used this remedy as an
application for earache, and it is effective as a
compress to ease painful joints. It is antispasmodic
and sedative, and valuable for spasmodic pains such
as neuralgia, colic and menstrual pains.

Melilot has a beneficial effect on the circulation,
and is considered by some authorities to be a
valuable anti-thrombotic agent.

15.

MINT
(Mentha)

The mints are native of European and Mediterranean
countries, some varieties being introduced into
Britain by the Romans. 'If one were to enumerate
completely all the virtues, varieties and names of
mints, one would be able to say how many fish are
swimming in the Red Sea'. So wrote a monk in the
ninth century.

With reference to headaches we are concerned
with only three species: Peppermint (*Mentha
piperita*), Spearmint (*Mentha viridis*) and Pennyroyal
(*Mentha pulegium*).

Peppermint tea, taken hot and frequently, is a
pleasant drink with the familiar flavour of oil of
Peppermint, and is a good remedy for headaches
which are the result of digestive or gall-bladder
disorders. They may be associated with bilious colic,
flatulence and a distended abdomen. An infusion
may be made by steeping four or five whole leaves

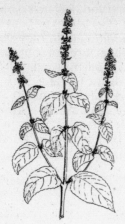

Mint

(fresh or dried) in a teacupful of boiling water for five minutes, being sure to keep it closely covered. Take this after meals, once or twice daily. This tea may also benefit headaches associated with nasal catarrh, when there is pain across the forehead with pain in or behind the eyes. It can also be helpful in affording relief in a nervous headache.

Peppermint leaves, infused briefly in warm water, are recommended as a compress for migraine and neuralgia, also for pains in the joints, the menthol present in the oil having an analgesic effect. The oil of Peppermint has an antispasmodic effect and acts as a powerful stimulant on secretion of bile.

Spearmint, of which Gerard said: 'The smell rejoiceth the heart of man' is the familiar culinary mint, which once planted in the garden will grow profusely. An infusion will ease vomiting and nausea, and the associated headache. Infuse for ten minutes, and drink a small wineglassful as required. The leaves may also be applied as a compress to the forehead.

Pennyroyal is a less pleasant mint, but was valued by Dioscorides and by Pliny, who praised its virtues in a number of disorders. It has been found effective for headaches with giddiness, or for headaches with a feeling of pain in bones, especially across the forehead. The dose is a small teacupful taken warm at frequent intervals until relief is felt. A hot infusion will promote perspiration in colds. Pennyroyal tea is an old remedy for delayed periods, so should not be taken during pregnancy.

16.

MISTLETOE
(Viscum album)

Known for its association with the Christmas festival, Mistletoe is revered by herbal practitioners for its sedative and antispasmodic properties. It is valuable

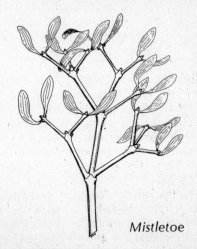

Mistletoe

for headaches and migraine which are due to hypertension (high blood pressure). Recent research has shown this remedy to be a safe hypotensive, having a relaxing action on the blood vessels, and is therefore used for arteriosclerosis and raised blood pressure.

The young leafy twigs, without berries, are used in the dried state, chopped, and prepared as a cold infusion: 25g (1 oz.) to ½ litre (1 pint) cold water, soaked overnight. Take a wineglassful on rising, mid-afternoon and at bedtime. This tea may be taken alone for headaches and migraine or – perhaps even more beneficially – may be combined in equal parts with Lime flower tea as a regular drink for high blood pressure, or for heart complaints of nervous origin such as palpitation. The leaves, infused for a few minutes in hot water, will relieve the pains of gout or rheumatism when applied as a compress.

17.

MOTHERWORT
(Leonurus cardiaca)

A member of the *Labiatae* – a Natural Order containing about 2,500 species – as are the Mints, Wood Betony, Lavender and Rosemary, Motherwort possesses the square stems and two-lipped flowers which signify plants of this group. The one British species grows on waste ground and in hedgerows, and was probably introduced into this country as it is native to Europe.

This remedy, which is sedative and antispasmodic, is valuable for headaches which occur at the menstrual period, especially when the period is unduly light, giving rise to a dull heavy headache on top of the head or across the forehead. There may be

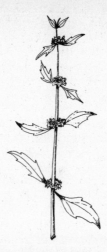

Motherwort

tension in the muscles at the back of the neck, or pain in the lower abdomen.

The normal infusion may be made, the dose being a wineglassful after meals. If this type of headache is experienced with every period it would be advisable to begin the herbal tea about one week before the period is due and continue until the period has been cleared.

Motherwort is a valuable heart remedy, particularly during convalescence, when associated with nervous symptoms such as palpitation, or in general debility.

18

PASSION FLOWER
(Passiflora incarnata)

A beautiful climbing plant which is native to America and has impressive large pale flowers with purple centres, *Passiflora incarnata* is one of 400 species. It was discovered by Spanish explorers and missionaries who gave it its name because of the supposed likeness of part of its flower to the crown of thorns.

This remedy is antispasmodic, sedative and anodyne, and is excellent for nervous headaches and for headaches with neuralgia. Indeed, its soothing effect on most nervous states affecting heart, stomach and menstruation has been found most beneficial. It is singularly successful in palpitation of

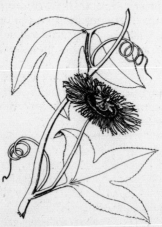

Passion Flower

nervous origin and for sleeplessness due to worry or anxiety.

This remedy should be prepared by adding 30-50g (about 1½ oz.) to 1 litre (2 pints) cold water, bringing gently to the boil, simmering for one minute, removing from heat and allowing to stand for ten minutes. Strain, and take a teacupful when required for a headache, or three times daily: on rising, at mid-afternoon and on retiring at night. Taken regularly at bedtime it will be conducive to peaceful sleep. Passion flower can be of considerable help during the menopause when it is accompanied by headaches, anxiety, palpitation and symptoms of indigestion.

19.

ROSEMARY
(Rosemarinus officinalis)

One of the best-known herbal remedies for headaches, a tea may be made by infusing 25g (1 oz.) of the herb in 1 litre (2 pints) of boiling water and allowing it to stand for ten minutes, or by infusing one teaspoonful of the crushed leaves in a teacupful of boiling water. Do not allow any steam to escape. The dose is a small teacupful, cool, when required for a headache, before each meal if there is liver malfunction, or after meals as a general tonic.

Rosemary exerts effect on the digestive system, improving secretion of bile and gastric juices, and is beneficial in all nervous disorders. It is a fine remedy for both a nervous headache and one due to gastric trouble, is used by the herbal practitioner for high blood pressure, as a heart tonic, and for a variety of nerve conditions. A wineglassful taken at bedtime will help induce sleep, especially if a warm bath containing a cupful of strong infusion is taken just

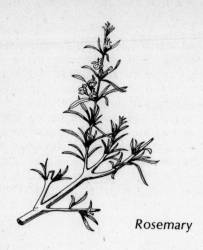

Rosemary

before retiring.

Rosemary has been valued throughout the ages, being regarded by the Romans as a sacred herb, bound in wreaths around the heads of Greek students to help combat brain-fatigue – recent experiments have proved the validity of external application for this condition – and is now proved to have antiseptic and anti-rheumatic properties. The plant contains 1 per cent-2 per cent of an essential oil, which has been used in perfumery and which is also a valuable ingredient in liniment for rheumatism and allied conditions. This oil has five times more powerful an antiseptic value than carbolic acid. Rosemary has properties which are tonic and stimulating to hair growth and nourishment, the oil being a primary constituent of many proprietary shampoos and hair lotions.

This is a delightful bush to have in the garden, possessing a pleasant fragrance, producing blue flowers in April and May, and acting as an insect repellant.

20

RUE
(Ruta graveolens)

A plant which grows in southern Europe,
recommended by Hippocrates and by Pliny, Rue is a
native of the Balkan peninsula and temperate Asia
which has been cultivated in western Europe for
several hundred years. It has greyish glaucous leaves,
which may be irritating to sensitive skins, and
curiously constructed yellowish flowers. Known as
the 'Herb of Grace' it had an almost magical
reputation as a cure for many conditions: for
improving eyesight, for nervous ailments and
nervous indigestion, a remedy to protect against
infection, to encourage or ease painful periods, and
numerous other conditions.

It is used successfully for headaches which result

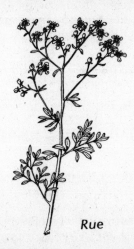

Rue

from eyestrain; the infusion may be prepared by adding one teaspoonful of the herb to a teacupful of boiling water and allowing to stand for ten minutes. When it is cool, take one tablespoonful to relieve a headache, or take three times daily. If strained through a fine cloth the infusion may be used as an eye lotion, diluted with equal parts of water. If combined with Scullcap and Valerian in equal parts, 25g (1 oz.) of the mixture to $\frac{1}{2}$ litre (1 pint) of boiling water, a tablespoonful dose taken between meals will afford relief in nervous headaches, giddiness and palpitation.

Rue contains about 0.1 per cent essential oil and – amongst other substances – the constituent rutin, which strengthens blood vessels, bones, nails and teeth. It has been found very beneficial for a number of women's ailments, but should not be taken during pregnancy.

This herb belongs to a Natural Order of which many species are aromatic and which includes the citrus plants, oranges and lemons. It has been discussed by many writers, praised by herbalists, and referred to several times by Shakespeare, who links it more than once with Rosemary:

> Reverend Sirs,
> For you there's rosemary and rue; these keep
> Seeming and savour all the winter long;
> Grace and remembrance be to you both.

21.

ST JOHN'S WORT
(Hypericum perforatum)

A common plant, one of the eleven British species of *Hypericum*, St John's Wort grows in woodlands and hedgerows, an erect branched plant up to about

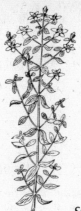

St John's Wort

50 cm (18 inches) in height, its bright yellow flowers gleam in the hedgerows during July and August. It includes 0.1 per cent essential oil and 10 per cent astringents among its constituents.

This remedy is sedative, and is effective in headaches with excitability, hysteria, neuralgia, especially such symptoms occurring at the menopause, for a heavy feeling in the head, perhaps with brain-fag, or with a throbbing on top of the head.

Two tablespoonsful of the normal infusion may be taken three times daily, or more frequently to relieve the symptoms mentioned above. Its astringent qualities have made this a widely-used remedy for many conditions for affecting the urinary system and the lungs, and for diarrhoea and dysentery. It has been found useful for enuresis – bedwetting – and for this a small teacupful of the infusion should be taken at bedtime. It is also used externally for wounds and bruises, burns, scalds, blisters and abrasions, for which either the infusion may be used or the fresh flowers steeped and heated gently in olive oil. St John's Wort was the main ingredient in an oil used by the Crusaders for their wounds.

Recent research has shown this plant to have a good effect on the secretion of bile and on basic metabolism, and that it will stimulate the appetite.

22.

SCULLCAP
(Scutellaria lateriflora)

A small plant with pale blue flowers which grows abundantly in America, this herb is a fine remedy for headaches of nervous origin, for a dull headache with aching eyes, or for a headache due to coughing. It is a valuable medicine for restlessness and irritability, excitability with twitching muscles, and is used extensively by the herbal practitioner in

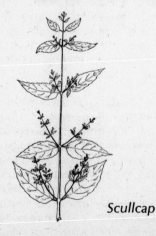

Scullcap

combination with other nervines for a wide range of conditions. Many authorities claim it to be the finest remedy for all nerve disorders ever discovered, and this may certainly be true.

It may be taken alone as an infusion – the warm infusion is more quickly effective and exerts its action more diffusively – or combined with other herbs in infusion, or may be used as a tincture alone or with other tinctures. The dose of the infusion is a small teacupful night and morning, or as required for a headache, regularly at bedtime for insomnia, and the dose of the tincture is five to ten drops in a little water. Combined with an equal quantity of Vervain (*Verbena officinalis*) a wineglassful of the normal infusion taken three times daily will quickly relieve headaches and general nervous irritability. Taken warm at bedtime it soothes and calms, reducing restlessness and helping to restore good sleep when the insomnia is due to mental exhaustion.

The herbal practitioner uses this remedy combined with cardiac agents for some heart conditions.

23.

VALERIAN
(*Valeriana officinalis*)

A migraine remedy, Valerian is one of the British members of an Order which grows in temperate regions in Europe, South America and northern India. Many of the plants are aromatic, the most notable being the Spikenard mentioned in the scriptures. The name Valerian is reputedly derived from the Latin *valere* 'to be in health'. It was recommended by Pliny as a treatment for nervous spasms, and was known as 'All-heal' in mediaeval

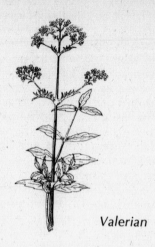

Valerian

times. *Valeriana officinalis* contains 1 per cent of volatile oil, valerianic acid, a number of minerals, and is rich in silica.

The plant is attractive with its inflorescence of pink flowers blooming from June to August, and is found along river banks, in damp areas, or on old walls. It is faintly perfumed, but its main odour is residual in the root, which is the part used. The smell of the root, which increases with age or with drying, may be the reason for the name 'Phu' by which it is believed to have been known to Galen. Cats have a liking for this smell, and will express their pleasure in transports of ecstasy.

Valerian is sedative, nervine, mildly anodyne, and is used by the herbal practitioner for a wide range of conditions: migraine, insomnia caused by nervous exhaustion, neuralgic pains, hysteria, and heart disorders of nervous origin, and it can be combined with other remedies for all types of nervous disorders.

A decoction may be prepared by adding 25g

(1 oz.) to 1 litre ($\frac{1}{2}$ pint) cold water, heating gently to just below boiling point and maintaining the temperature for ten minutes. The dose is two tablespoonsful three times daily before meals, or at bedtime. It would be advisable to add a little honey and some pleasant herb such as Peppermint (which reinforces the action of Valerian), Vervain or Balm. It may be combined in equal parts with Scullcap, Vervain, and adding half the quantity of Peppermint and Gentian. Infuse in the normal manner, taking a tablespoonful before meals. Discontinue the Valerian after two or three weeks of regular dosing, and recommence after a few days.

24.

WOOD BETONY
(Betonica officinalis)

Wood betony has been used since the Greek civilization for headaches and for a variety of conditions. Proverbs extol its value: the Italians advised 'Sell your coat and buy Betony'. It has been widely used by physicians throughout the ages, was praised by Dioscorides and Galen, was one of the remedies cultivated in monastery gardens, is subject to modern research, and figures prominently in the herbalist's dispensary.

Wood Betony is used for headaches, anxiety, neuralgia, nervous migraine, liver and biliary disorders, gout and some forms of rheumatism, and for a wide range of symptoms affecting the head, especially in a patient of excitable disposition. A wineglassful of the infusion may be taken three or more times daily, or can be combined in equal parts with Scullcap, or prepared as a decoction which, it is claimed, will cure the worst kind of nervous

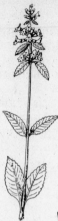

Wood Betony

headache. For this method add 50g (2 oz.) herb to 1 litre (2 pints) boiling water, simmer gently (covered) until reduced to ¾ litre (1½ pints). Cool, strain, and take a wineglassful three or four times daily regularly. The length of time necessary to continue taking this will depend entirely on the duration and intensity of the headaches. Attention may have to be paid to diet if there is no improvement.

The infusion may be taken for headaches which develop during a cold or chill, in which instance it could be combined with Elderflowers.

THERAPEUTIC INDEX

Anxiety Passion flower, Wood betony
Biliousness Chamomile, Gentian, Mint
Brain-fatigue Rosemary, St John's Wort
Catarrh Anemone, Mint
Children Chamomile
Colds Lime, Mint
Constipation Dandelion
Debility Gentian, Hops
Digestion Chamomile, Gentian, Hops, St John's Wort
Exhaustion Gentian, Hops
External application Hops, Lavender, Melilot, Mint, Mistletoe, St John's Wort
Flatulence Chamomile, Mint
Giddiness Lavender, Mint (Pennyroyal), Rue
Hair Rosemary
Headaches
  Dull Dandelion, Gentian, Lime, Scullcap
  Forehead Gentian, Mint, Motherwort
  Throbbing Chamomile (German), Melilot
  Top of head Anemone, Feverfew, Motherwort, St John's Wort
Heart Motherwort, Passion flower, Rosemary, Valerian
High Blood Pressure Lime, Melilot, Mistletoe
Hysteria Feverfew, St John's Wort, Valerian, Wood Betony
Indigestion Gentian, Lavender, Passion flower, Rosemary
Insomnia Anemone, Hops, Lime, Passion flower, Rosemary, Scullcap, Valerian
Irritability Chamomile (German), Hops, Scullcap

Kidneys Corn Silk, Couch Grass
Liver Dandelion, Couch Grass, Rosemary
Menopause Feverfew, Passion flower, St John's Wort
Menstruation Anemone, Chamomile, Feverfew, Melilot, Motherwort
Mental fatigue Anemone, Rosemary, Scullcap
Migraine Dandelion, Lavender, Lime, Mint, Mistletoe, Valerian, Wood Betony
Nausea Chamomile, Corn Silk, Gentian, Lime, Melilot, Mint
Nerves Motherwort, Passion flower, Rosemary, Rue, Scullcap, Valerian
Neuralgia Anemone, Hops, Lime, Melilot, Mint, Passion flower, St John's Wort, Valerian
Nightmares Chamomile, Hops
Palpitation Lavender, Mistletoe, Motherwort, Passion flower
Restlessness Chamomile, Hops, Scullcap
Rheumatism Rosemary
Tension Anemone, Chamomile, Hops, Lime
Urinary conditions Dandelion, Lime, St John's Wort